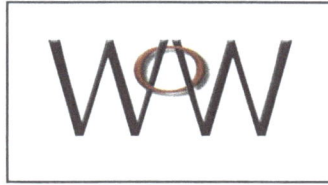

Choosing a
Career as a
Nurse-Midwife

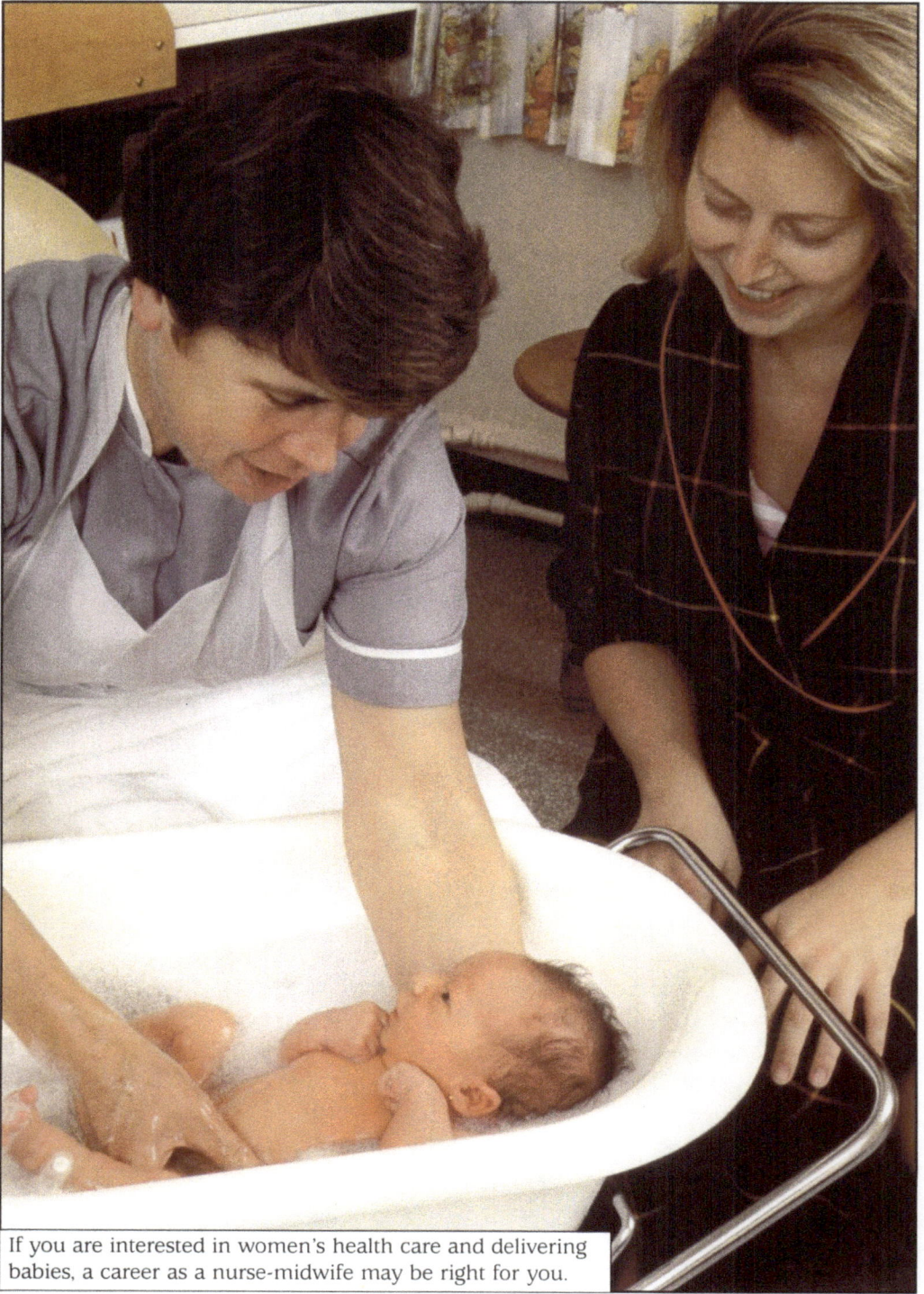

If you are interested in women's health care and delivering babies, a career as a nurse-midwife may be right for you.

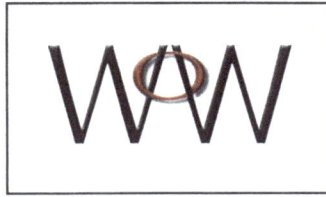

Choosing
a Career
as a
Nurse-Midwife

Jennifer Fields

The Rosen Publishing Group, Inc.
New York

To Simon

Published in 2001 by The Rosen Publishing Group, Inc.
29 East 21st Street, New York, NY 10010

First Edition

Library of Congress Cataloging-in-Publication Data

Fields, Jennifer.
Choosing a career as a nurse-midwife / by Jennifer Fields.—1st ed.
    p.   cm.—(The world of work)
Includes bibliographical references and index.
ISBN 978-1-4358-8672-8
1. Midwifery—Vocational guidance—Juvenile literature. 2. Nursing—Vocational guidance—Juvenile literature. [1. Midwives—Vocational guidance. 2. Vocational Guidance.] [DNLM: 1. Midwifery—Popular Works. 2. Career Choice—Popular Works. WQ 160 F462c 2000] I. Title. II. World of work (New York, N.Y.)
RG950 .F54 2000
618.2'0233—dc21   00-011988

Manufactured in the United States of America

Contents

Introduction

Michaele Wylde is a thirty-four-year-old woman who lives with her husband and two children in Brooklyn, New York. When she was pregnant with her first baby a few years ago, she knew she wanted to have her baby with a nurse-midwife. No other way would do.

Michaele says, "I heard from my friends that midwives spend more time with you. They have a more natural and less medical approach and I was very interested in natural childbirth." She liked the idea that her baby would be delivered with the help of someone who was less like a doctor, and more like a friend. Someone who would hold her hand and comfort her. She wanted someone who would be there with her throughout the entire process: preparing to have a baby, labor, and delivery.

"I like midwives because they treat you as a person rather than a bunch of symptoms. My midwife was personable, warm, and spent lots of time talking with me. My care was exceptional," she says. "I love my midwife. We even became good friends."

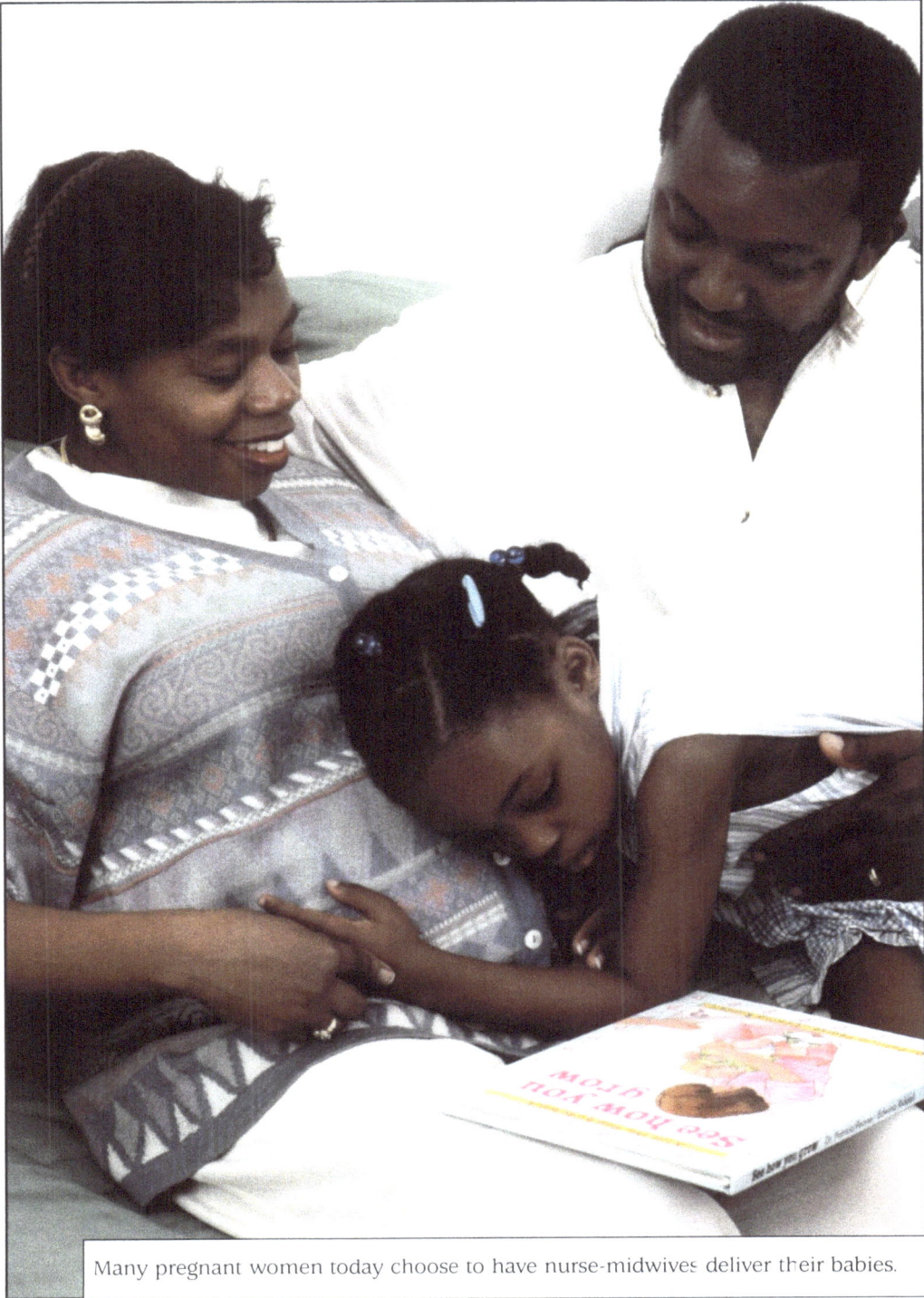

Many pregnant women today choose to have nurse-midwives deliver their babies.

Child Birth: A Family Affair

Michaele Wylde is like many women today. They know that childbirth can be scary and painful. They look to a nurse-midwife to provide health care that includes emotional support—a hand to hold. For hundreds of years, many societies considered childbirth a community event; some still do. Birthing was considered a very sacred and woman-centered experience.

Female friends and family members tended to women giving birth in their own homes. These women had also borne children, so they knew what to expect and how to be helpful. As experienced mothers, they offered a pregnant woman comfort during labor. They helped her deliver the baby, guiding her through labor, holding her hand, wiping her brow, and cleaning the new arrival. They stayed with her after the birth to cook for the family, teach the new mother how to feed the baby, and assist her while she adjusted to the demands of motherhood.

Nowadays, we tend to think of childbirth as clinical—happening in a hospital, supervised by a doctor, and aided by a nurse. You have probably seen television programs in which a woman in labor is rushed off to the hospital in an ambulance. One friend or family member keeps her company while other family and friends wait outside. After the woman has endured hours of labor, a doctor arrives to deliver the baby. Once the baby is welcomed into the world, a proud partner shares the big news with everyone who has gathered in the waiting room.

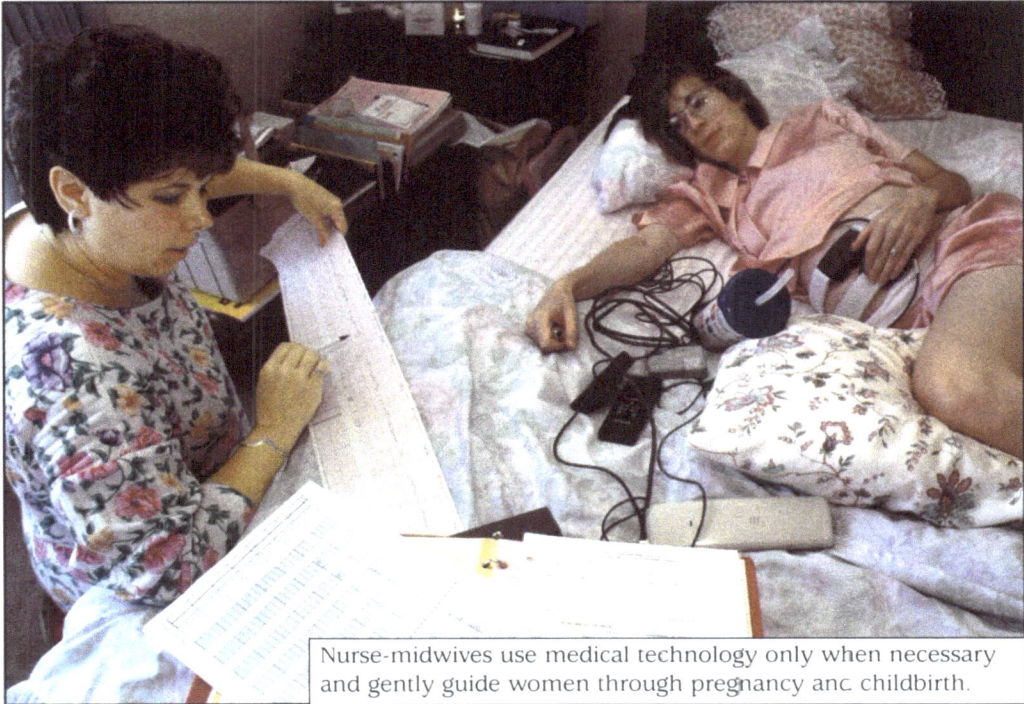
Nurse-midwives use medical technology only when necessary and gently guide women through pregnancy and childbirth.

One problem with this approach is that it tends to define pregnancy and childbirth as illnesses. Nurse-midwives want to put women at the center of birthing and treat delivery as a special event. Nurse-midwives view pregnancy and childbirth as natural and normal processes that require little intervention. They have access to medical technology, but use it only when absolutely necessary.

Nurse-midwives believe that women should be able to have their babies in a comfortable environment. Nurse-midwives stay with pregnant women throughout their entire labors, which can last many hours. They gently guide women through pregnancy and childbirth. They understand that childbirth can sometimes be scary and painful. They know that if they keep a woman in labor calm, the delivery will be easier.

9

1

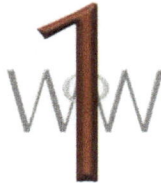

What Is a Nurse-Midwife?

The word midwife means "with woman." And indeed, that is one of the best ways to describe the work that nurse-midwives do: they are with women at one of the most exciting and sometimes frightening times of their lives. They care for women throughout their entire pregnancy and share in the moment of a new child coming into the world. A nurse-midwife is both a highly skilled professional and a comforting friend.

Early midwives were always women, and in many cases it was considered taboo for men to be present during birth. But that has all changed. Just as women now work in traditionally male fields such as medicine and law, men work in traditionally female fields like teaching and nursing. Currently, there are very few male nurse-midwives, but they do exist. Only one percent of the members of the American College of Nurse-Midwives (the national organization of nurse-midwives) are men. But the number is growing.

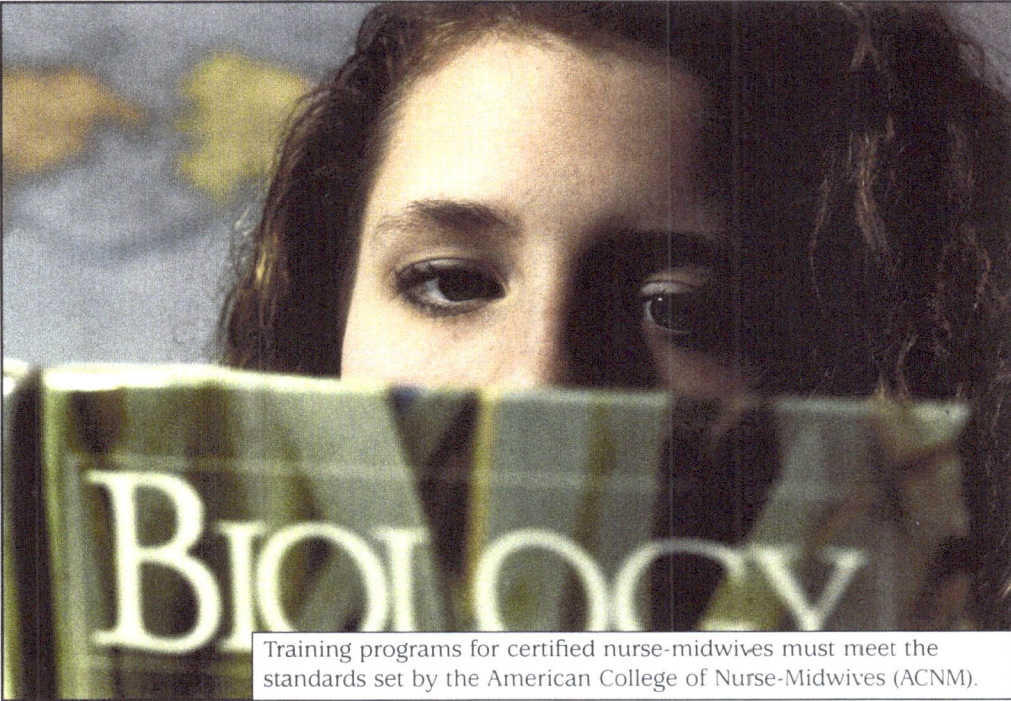

Training programs for certified nurse-midwives must meet the standards set by the American College of Nurse-Midwives (ACNM).

American College of Nurse-Midwives

All certified nurse-midwives meet the standards set forth by the American College of Nurse-Midwives (ACNM). These standards guarantee that all nurse-midwives receive the same training and possess the same qualifications. The ACNM offers guides, books, and magazines to help nurse-midwives keep up on new developments in the field. The ACNM also organizes annual conferences where nurse-midwives meet, discuss their work, and review developments in the field of women's health.

Like a doctor, a certified nurse-midwife has professional and moral duties to uphold. For that reason, the ACNM developed a code of ethics for nurse-midwives. This code highlights the obligations nurse-midwives owe their patients. The code guides the nurse-midwife during her practice. It also serves to clarify the goals and standards of nurse-midwives for patients, other medical professionals, and the general public.

Code of Ethics for Nurse-Midwives

✔ Nurse-midwifery exists for the good of women and their families. Nurse-midwives practice in accordance with the ACNM Philosophy and ACNM Standards for the Practice of Nurse-Midwifery.

✔ Nurse-midwives believe that childbearing and maturation are normal life processes. When intervention is indicated, it is integrated into care in a way that preserves the dignity of the woman and her family.

✔ Decisions regarding nurse-midwifery care require client participation in an ongoing negotiation process in order to develop a safe plan of care. This process considers cultural diversity, individual autonomy, and legal responsibilities.

✔ Nurse-midwives share professional information with their clients that leads to informed participation and consent. This sharing is done without coercion or deception.

✔ Nurse-midwives practice competently. They consult and refer when indicated by their professional scope of practice and/or personal limitations.

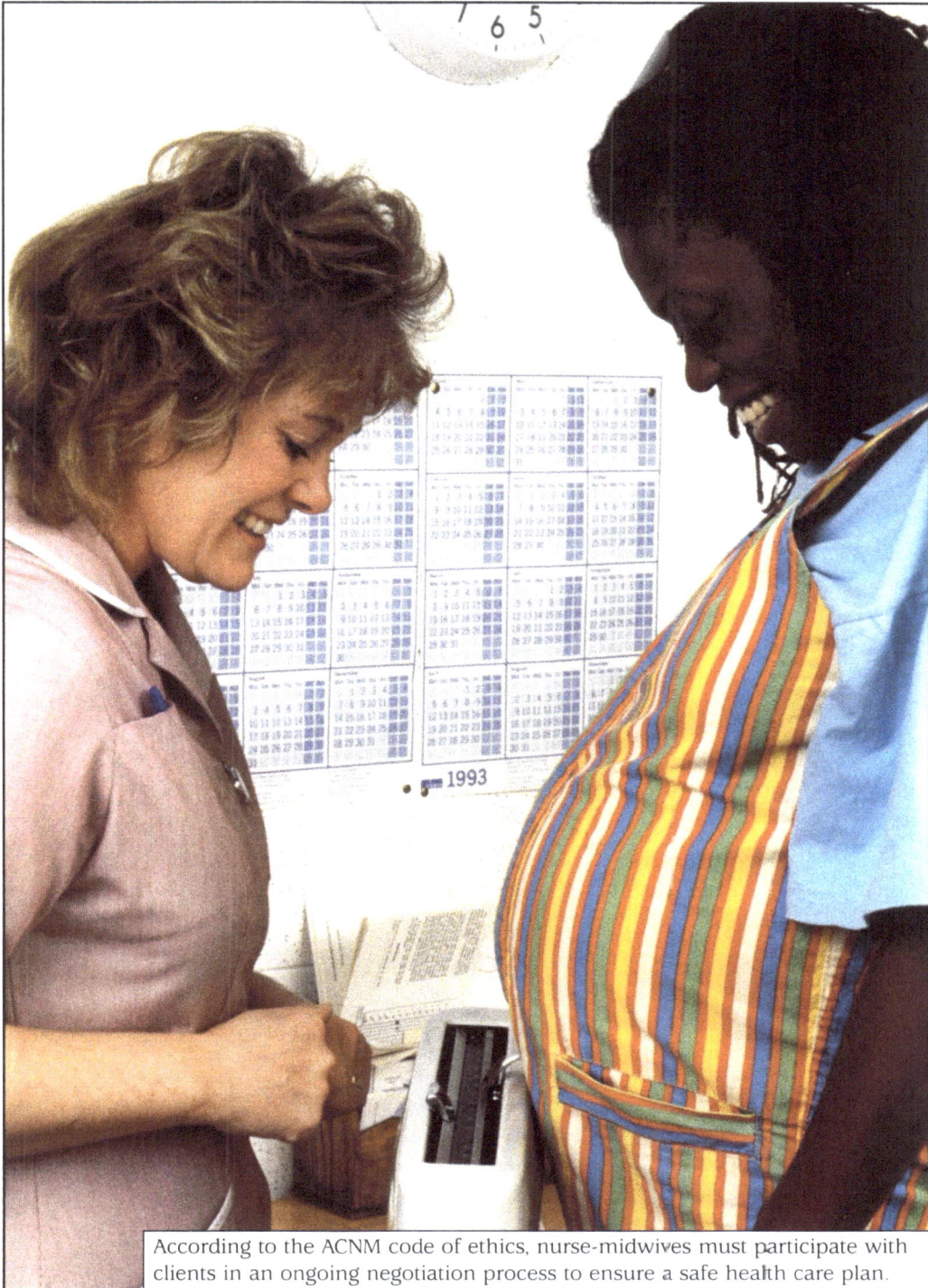

According to the ACNM code of ethics, nurse-midwives must participate with clients in an ongoing negotiation process to ensure a safe health care plan.

✔ Nurse-midwives provide care without discrimination based on race, religion, life-style, sexual orientation, socio-economic status, or nature of health problem.

✔ Nurse-midwives maintain confidentiality except when there is a clear, serious, and immediate danger or when mandated by law.

✔ Nurse-midwives take appropriate action to protect clients from harm when endangered by incompetent or unethical practices.

✔ Nurse-midwives interact respectfully with the people with whom they work and practice.

✔ Nurse-midwives participate in developing and improving the care of women and families through supporting the profession of nurse-midwifery, research, and the education of nurse-midwifery students and nurse-midwives.

✔ Nurse-midwives promote community, state, and national efforts such as public education and legislation, to ensure access to quality care and to meet the health needs of women and their families.

Nurse-Midwife Philosophy

Nurse-midwives hold certain beliefs about health care, women, and childbirth. Nurse-midwives feel that every person has a right to safe, satisfying health care. They believe that health care professionals should respect each client's cultural values. They encourage each patient to fully participate in his or her health care decisions.

They approach caring for their clients with a spirit of cooperation. According to the desires of the patient, they welcome the input of family, friends, or other medical providers. Nurse-midwives care for patients from pregnancy through to delivery. They encourage safe medical practices and intervene as little as possible. Nurse-midwives also actively promote health education for women.

2

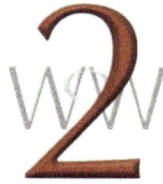

An Ancient Profession

Historians have noted that midwifery has existed throughout time and in many cultures. As women gave birth, they sought and received care from supportive friends and family. At an unknown point in human history, some experienced women were chosen as the wise women who should attend birth. This is how midwifery began.

During Greek and Roman times, midwives functioned as respected care providers for women. Soon qualifications for the practice of midwifery began to be established. For example, in ancient Greece a midwife was always a woman who had already borne children herself. This requirement was common to the practice of midwifery in many cultures and continues to exist in some societies.

The profession of midwifery continued without major changes for many centuries, even through the Dark and Middle Ages. In their practices, midwives routinely used herbs and potions as we now often use factory-produced drugs or pharmaceuticals. Generally, the midwives of these past centuries learned by starting as apprentices. They observed

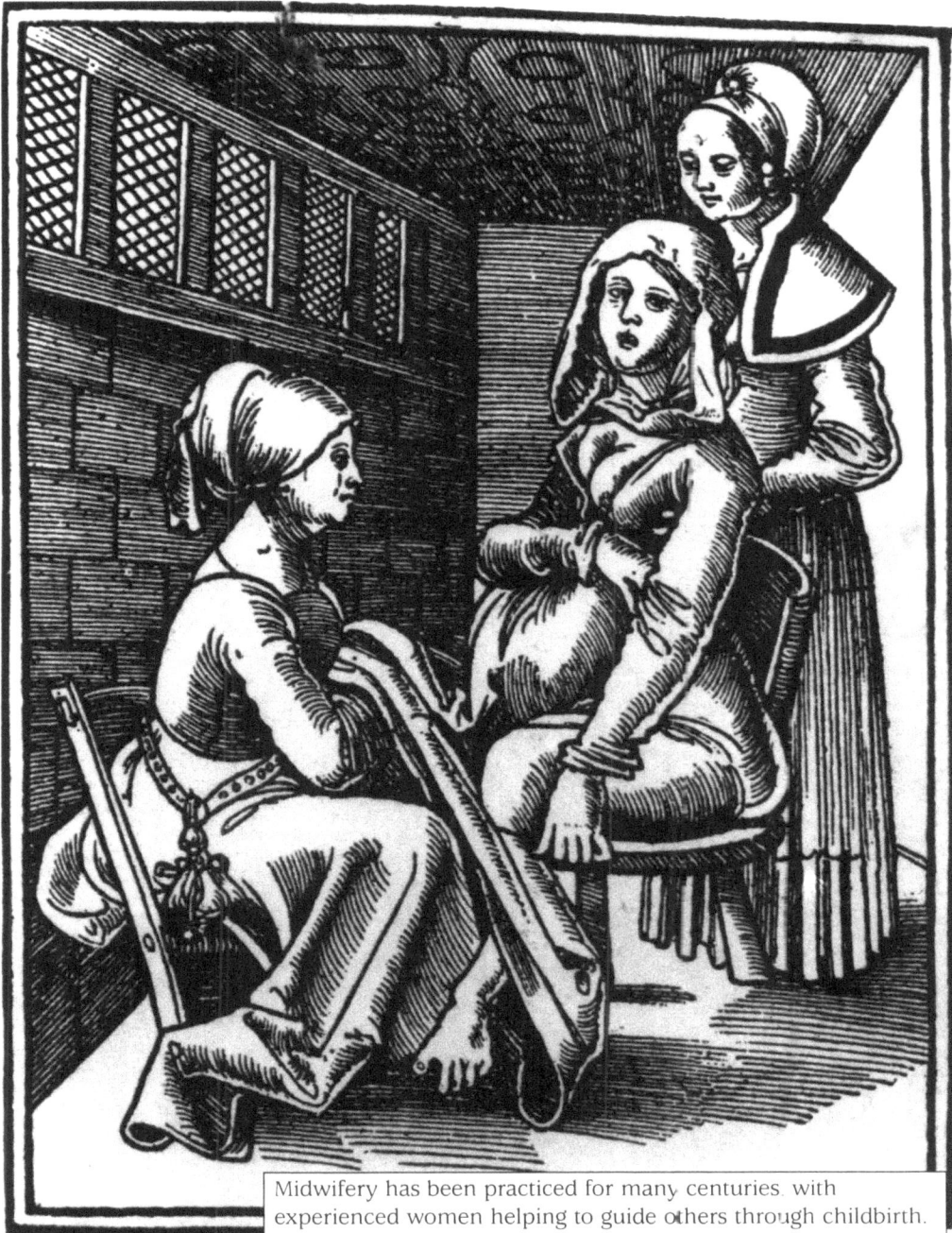

Midwifery has been practiced for many centuries, with experienced women helping to guide others through childbirth.

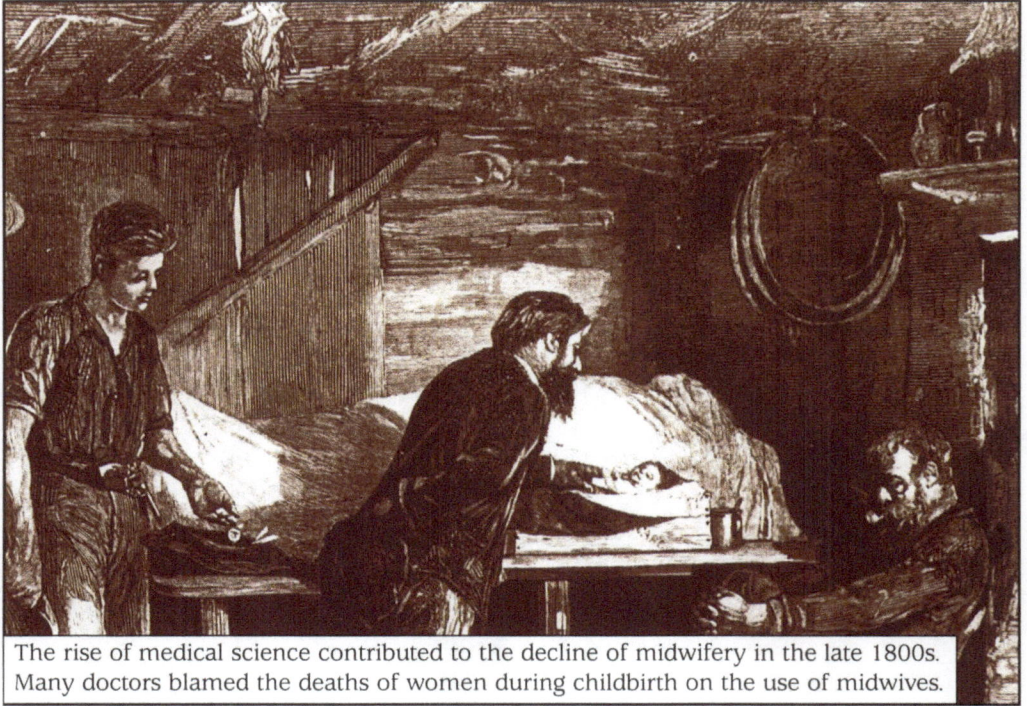

The rise of medical science contributed to the decline of midwifery in the late 1800s. Many doctors blamed the deaths of women during childbirth on the use of midwives.

the practices of more experienced midwives. These midwives handed down skills and information from generation to generation.

In the United States

"As a culture we really have to figure out how we got so afraid of birth and why, of all places in the world, we got rid of midwives here," observes Ina May Gaskin, one of the founders and the current president of the Midwives' Alliance of North America (MANA).

Although midwives have practiced for centuries, in the United States starting in the late 1800s, women used midwives less and less. A major factor that contributed to this decline was the rise of medical science. The development of two branches of medicine, obstetrics and gynecology, heavily influenced the way many people today think of pregnancy and childbirth.

Obstetricians are medical doctors who specialize in the care of pregnant women and deliver babies. Gynecologists are also medical doctors. They specialize in women's reproductive health, but they do not deliver babies. In 1888, these two groups of physicians joined together and formed the American Association of Obstetricians and Gynecologists (AAOG).

At that time, the AAOG was a strong organization of men, and as such, they possessed more political power and social influence than women. The group emphasized that childbirth was a complicated and dangerous process. Many of these doctors blamed the deaths of women during childbirth on the use of midwives.

The AAOG ignored the possibility that other factors affecting women, such as poor nutrition, lack of access to health care, and illness during pregnancy, might also cause these deaths. Instead, they argued that doctors, using instruments, drugs, and surgery, should manage childbirth. Only doctors could make sure a pregnant woman and her child would remain healthy and safe. They claimed that midwives did not have the proper training to deliver babies and began to convince people that childbirth should be doctor-supervised. Further, they argued that childbirth needed to happen in a controlled environment, such as a hospital.

In the late nineteenth century, formal university training programs did not yet exist for midwives. As a result, midwives had difficulty organizing into a powerful group, like the AAOG. For this reason, they lacked the means to publicly counter the claims doctors made about the safety of their methods.

Nurse-Midwives

The history of nurse-midwifery in the United States begins in Kentucky. In the early 1920s, a nurse named Mary Breckinridge founded the Frontier Nursing Service. Her goal was to provide health care to people in the remote areas of the Appalachian Mountains by sending nurses on horseback to see their patients.

Breckinridge had also trained to be a midwife in England. Breckinridge thought a system of midwives could serve women in the United States. In rural areas, many women and children died because they did not receive proper prenatal care and lacked medical help during delivery. She hoped that bringing midwives to poor women living in these areas would reduce the number of deaths during childbirth.

In 1929, Breckinridge invited British midwives to come to the United States to serve patients and train nurses. They were the first nurse-midwives in the United States. Along with the others from the Frontier Nursing Service, they were able to lower the number of deaths in childbirth. The midwives taught rural women and their families about proper hygiene and nutrition.

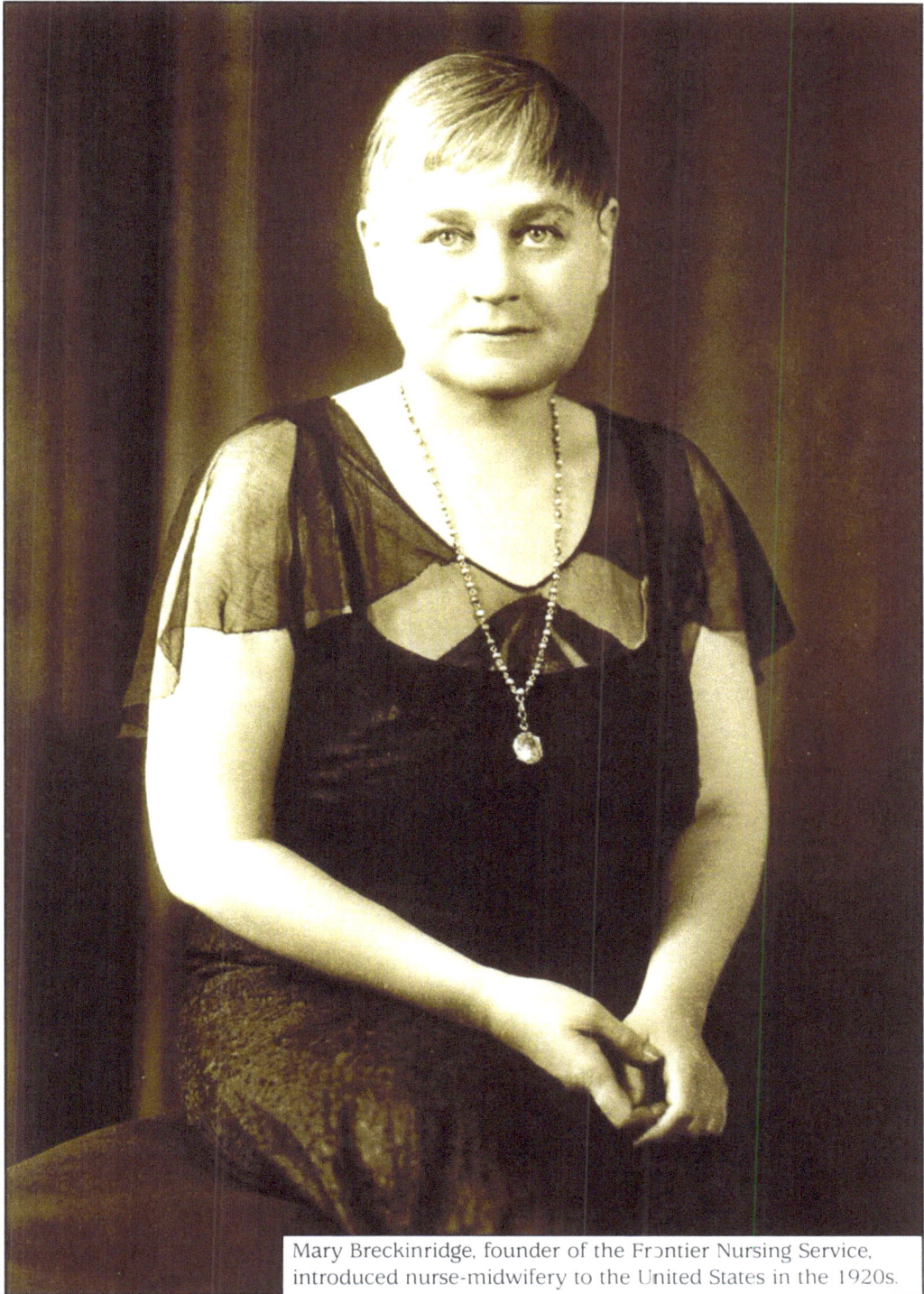

Mary Breckinridge, founder of the Frontier Nursing Service, introduced nurse-midwifery to the United States in the 1920s.

The use of midwives in these areas succeeded; the number of deaths of women and children in childbirth dropped. Dr. Louis Dublin conducted a study of the first 1,000 births attended by nurse-midwives in this area. He reported that no deaths of mothers occurred due to pregnancy or labor.

The Frontier Nursing Service opened The Frontier Graduate School of Midwifery in 1939. Mary Breckinridge ran the school until she died in 1965. It continues to operate today. These midwives provided health care for poor and rural women who would have had little access to health care otherwise.

More colleges and universities began to develop nurse-midwife training programs. The American College of Nurse-Midwifery was chartered in 1955. In 1969, this organization combined with the American Association of Nurse-Midwives to form the American College of Nurse-Midwives. Today, the ACNM continues to set the standards for teaching and practicing nurse-midwifery.

Nurse-midwifery is a relatively new development. They are midwives who are also trained nurses. With this additional schooling and experience they seem more legitimate not only to physicians but also to lawmakers. As a result, nurse-midwifery is a legally recognized profession in every state.

Direct-Entry Midwives

Today, some people continue to practice midwifery although they do not have a nursing degree or formal nursing training. They are direct-entry midwives

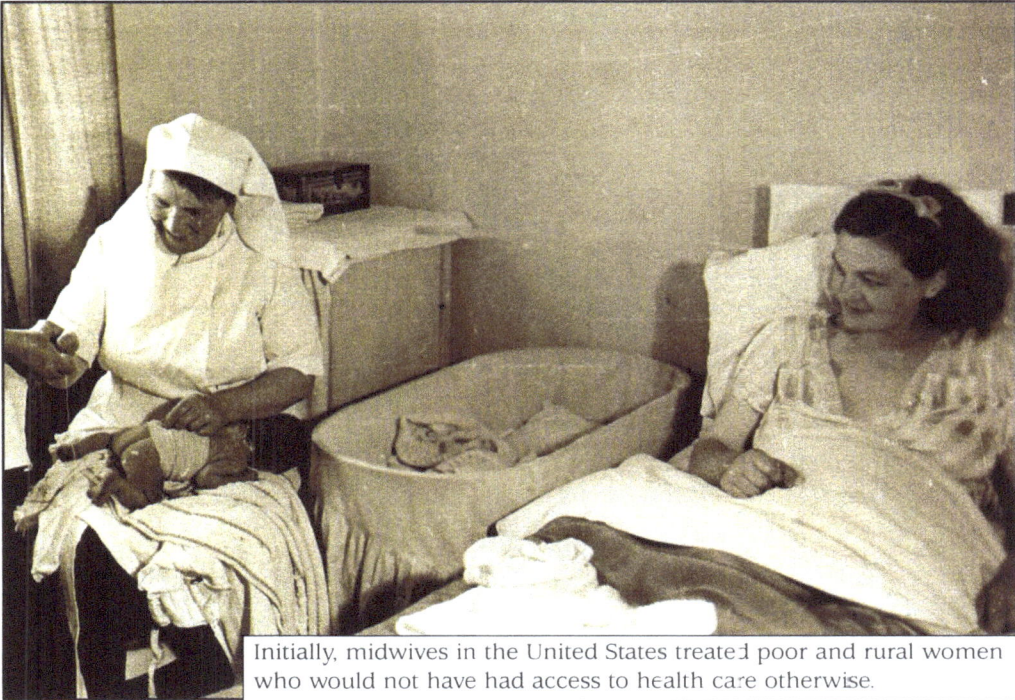

Initially, midwives in the United States treated poor and rural women who would not have had access to health care otherwise.

(DEM). Direct-entry midwives more closely resemble the earlier models of midwives, when women learned to deliver babies by watching others. Nowadays, both men and women interested in direct-entry midwifery train with experienced midwives. They sit in on prenatal examinations, births, and home-visits. Sometimes these midwives begin as childbirth assistants or childbirth educators. (See the section on related professions in chapter 5.)

In 1976, Ina May Gaskin, considered the mother of modern midwifery, published *Spiritual Midwifery*. In the book, she discusses her experience as a midwife using home-birth stories, black-and-white photography, and information on caring for women during pregnancy and childbirth. Gaskin went on to describe birth as a spiritual event. This was a revolutionary idea at a time when the ancient profession of direct-entry or

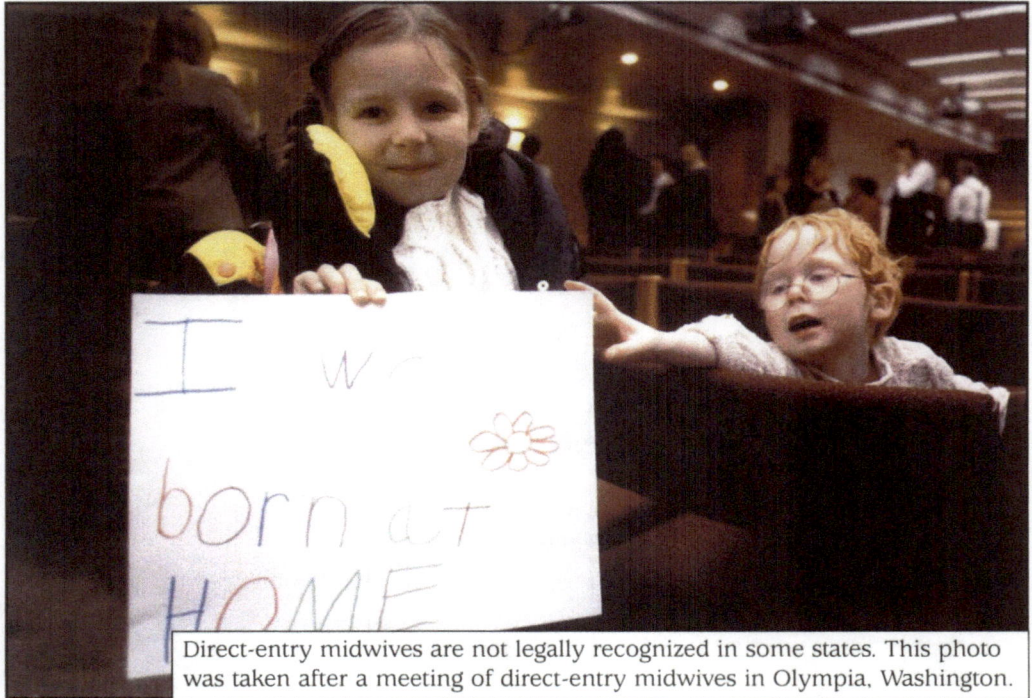

Direct-entry midwives are not legally recognized in some states. This photo was taken after a meeting of direct-entry midwives in Olympia, Washington.

"lay" midwifery had all but died out under pressure from physicians' groups.

After learning from other midwives, apprentices usually decide to become midwives themselves. This route can take about two years. Some states may register and license these types of midwives to assure people that they are qualified and competent. In other states, this type of midwifery is illegal. You have to find out what is allowed where you live, and you can do that by contacting the midwifery associations listed at the end of the book.

The fact that direct-entry midwives are not legally recognized in every state does not mean that their work is any less important or less valued. Direct-entry midwives are very important. This type of midwifery allows compassionate, hard-working people who are interested in delivering healthy babies to practice midwifery without attending nursing school.

Two Paths

In addition to the legal considerations, there are many other differences between nurse-midwives and direct-entry midwives. Nurse-midwives usually, but not always, practice in hospitals and doctors' offices. They stay connected to a doctor who can take over in an emergency. This association with a doctor often determines where a nurse-midwife works.

Direct-entry midwives, unlike nurse-midwives, attend births in family homes or in birth centers. Very few direct-entry midwives work in hospitals. As a result, they can more freely use alternative treatments. These treatments might include massage and herbal therapies for pain relief.

Almost all direct-entry midwives are in business for themselves. They might work longer hours but have more flexibility than a nurse-midwife. Direct-entry midwives set their own hours, so they can usually spend more time with women during routine visits and through childbirth.

Nurse-midwives usually work for hospitals or doctors. They tend to make more money and have regular hours and vacation time, but they have less say in what they do. Nurse-midwives may also be limited in the treatments they offer because they must abide by the policies of a hospital or doctor's practice.

Throughout its history, the profession of nurse-midwifery has withstood and overcome many obstacles. It has also gained acceptance by other health professionals. The profession continues to grow because of the unique type of care and support nurse-midwives provide women and their families.

Ask Yourself

Certainly, the history of nurse-midwifery shows that people can think of pregnancy and childbirth in very different ways. How you think pregnant women should be cared for will influence your decision to become a nurse-midwife. Here are some questions to ask yourself: Do I believe that pregnancy is natural and should not be treated like an illness? Do I believe that births should be family-centered? Am I calm in tense situations? Do I have a deep caring for the well-being of women and their families?

3

Becoming a Nurse-Midwife

In the first year of most nurse-midwifery programs, students learn about labor, birth, and caring for a newborn baby. This material is very general. Before you can study nurse-midwifery in-depth, it is important to have this overview.

You will also study the history of midwifery. We have already discussed a little of the history here. You will also learn some of the ethical questions people studying midwifery have faced in the past and still deal with today. For instance, it is important to know and respect the birth traditions of different cultures. Nurse-midwives care for women whose religious beliefs, cultural values, and ethnic backgrounds may vary from their own. It is important to understand other people's beliefs about birth and to treat each client respectfully.

Also early in nurse-midwifery study, you will gain a basic understanding of the body and how it works. You will learn all about women's health. You will study the basics of how a fetus develops inside a woman's body, and the effect a woman's eating habits have on the growth of the fetus. You will

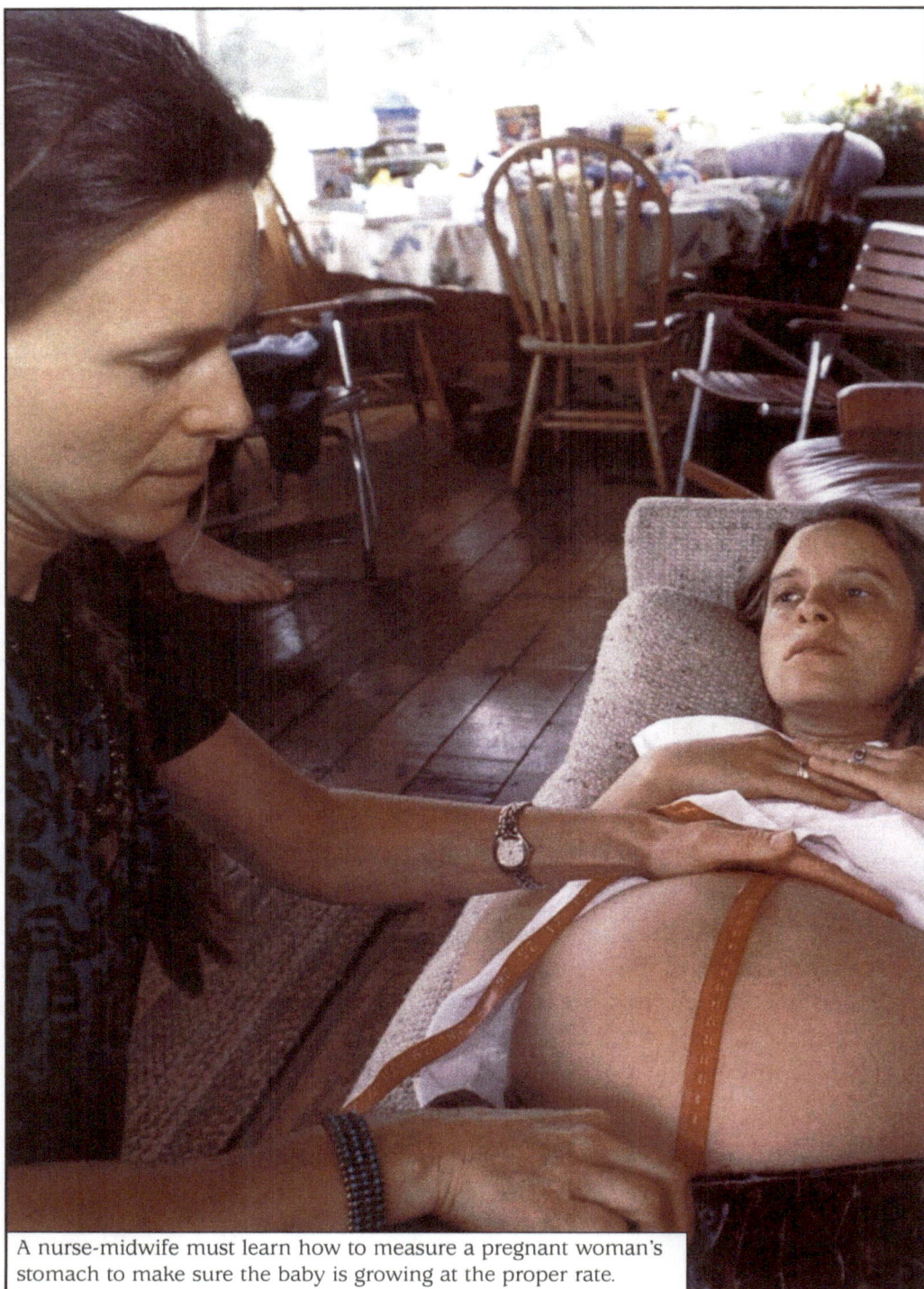

A nurse-midwife must learn how to measure a pregnant woman's stomach to make sure the baby is growing at the proper rate.

begin to understand the specific needs of a woman's body at every stage of pregnancy, including her emotional needs. You will also learn the impact of certain things like stress, smoking, drinking alcohol, and illness on a pregnancy.

As schooling continues, you will study the more technical aspects of being a nurse-midwife. You will learn how to take blood for tests and how to read the results. You will study the way to perform regular routine exams for women. These exams might include tests for cancer, pregnancy, and infections, as well as breast exams.

Of course, you will also study how to examine a pregnant woman. This includes measuring a pregnant woman's stomach to make sure the baby is growing at the proper rate, screening pregnant women for infections, monitoring the baby's heart rate, and checking the mother's blood pressure.

You will learn about all the equipment and tools that nurse-midwives use, like ultrasound machines that deliver pictures of the baby. These pictures allow nurse-midwives to check for any problems and can even detect the sex of the baby. You will also be taught how to administer pain medication. You will even learn how to support a woman in labor.

As you become a more advanced student, you will study the different complications that might arise during pregnancy, and how to manage them. You will also learn which complications might require the assistance of a doctor. You will study possible illnesses and abnormalities that babies can develop before they are born.

You will learn how to provide patients with psychological guidance and support. Nurse-midwives sometimes need to respond to family crises such as abuse or illegal drug use. Also, as much as nurse-midwives deal with birth, they may also witness death. This is a reality for all health care professionals, including nurse-midwives. Instruction in counseling will help prepare you to help your patients.

Before you know it, you will be ready to spend the last year of your study as an apprentice. You will work with other nurse-midwives in their private practices or in hospitals. You will get to observe for yourself what they do everyday.

Preparing for a Nurse-Midwifery Program

If you are planning to be a nurse-midwife, you can start preparing for your career as early as high school. Of course, admissions counselors at nurse-midwifery programs will look for good grades. They will also review your school transcripts to see that you took science classes like chemistry, biology, or physiology.

Admissions counselors also prefer candidates who have volunteer experience related to childbirth. Think about participating in extracurricular activities; this will demonstrate your ability to balance several tasks at once. Further, take on a leadership role at school; leadership is an important part of being a nurse-midwife.

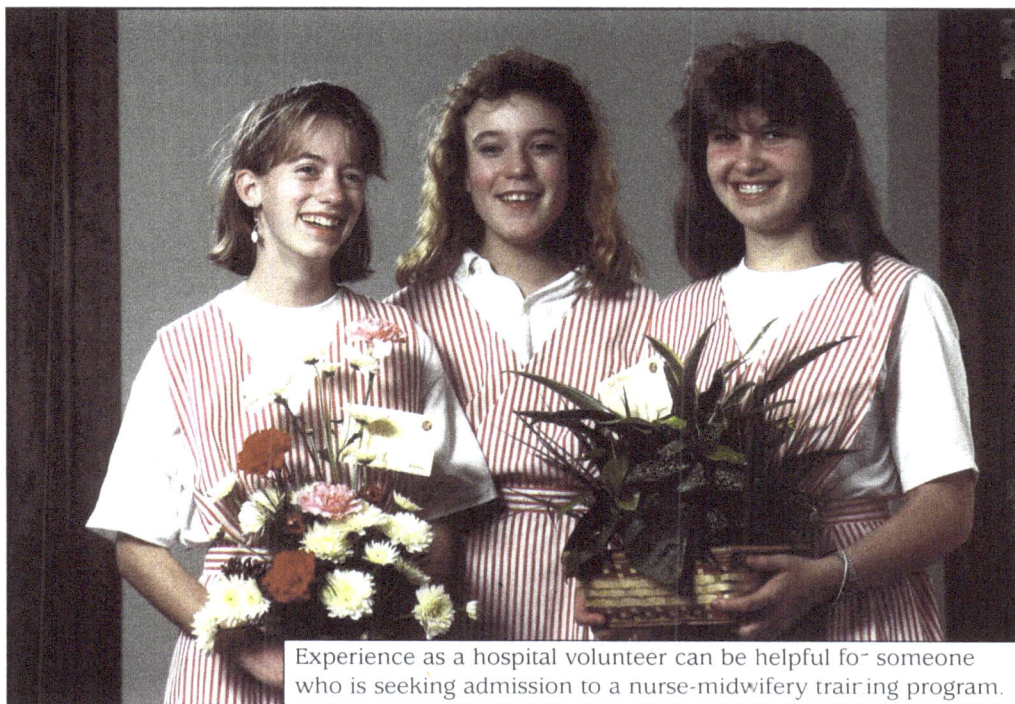

Experience as a hospital volunteer can be helpful for someone who is seeking admission to a nurse-midwifery training program.

You might consider attending workshops and conferences related to midwifery. You should also think about learning another language. Many of your patients may not speak English. By knowing another language, such as Spanish, you can more easily put your non-English speaking patients at ease.

A Growing Field

Today, there are fifty nurse-midwifery education programs in the United States approved by the American College of Nurse-Midwives. Most of these programs offer bachelor's and master's degrees. Only about 5 percent of these programs offer doctoral degrees.

About two-thirds of nurse-midwives have a master's degree. There are also nontraditional

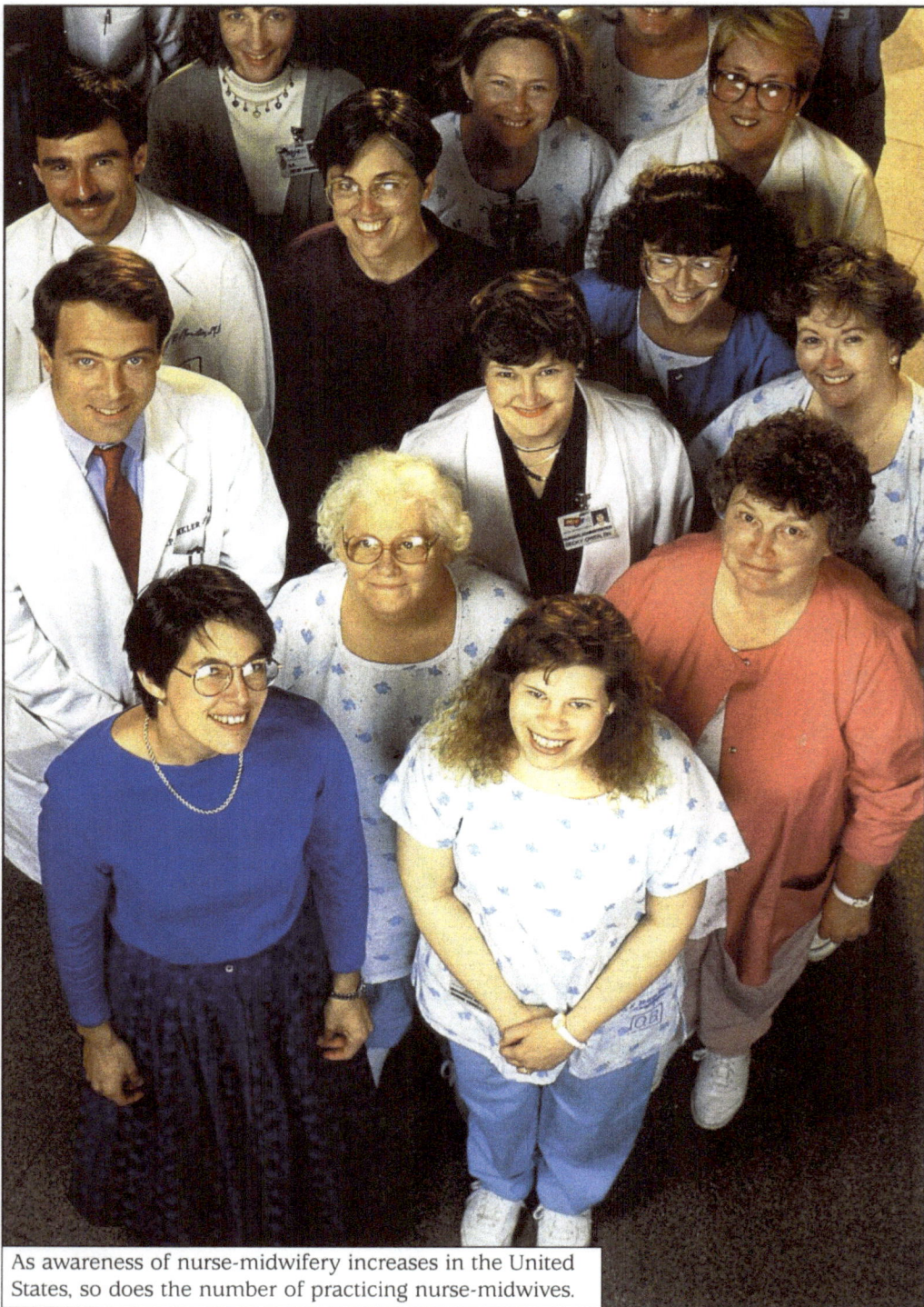

As awareness of nurse-midwifery increases in the United States, so does the number of practicing nurse-midwives.

ways to earn your degree such as distance learning programs. In these programs, students living in remote areas, far from any college or university, use a computer to study and take classes. Almost 100 nurse-midwives use these programs every year.

The ACNM currently has more than 6,300 members. Of that number, about 5,000 are in clinical practice. The rest are students, teachers, and retired midwives.

Every year, about 400 nurse-midwives pass the national certification exam. That number is steadily increasing. Each year, in this country, certified nurse-midwives deliver almost 200,000 babies, mostly in hospitals. That accounts for almost 5 percent of all births in the United States.

Awareness of midwifery in the United States is on the rise. Preference for in-hospital, nurse-midwife-assisted births in the United States grew from about 20,000 in 1975 to almost 239,090 in 1996. Currently, approximately 30,000 women each year give birth in planned home-births.

Interestingly, of all visits to nurse-midwives, almost 80 percent are for general and preventative care. Nurse-midwives also see women who are not pregnant. Women visit for annual reproductive health or gynecological visits. Nurse-midwives, on average, spend almost an hour with a new patient and about a half an hour with return patients. There are now approximately 10,000 midwives, both direct-entry and nurse-midwives, practicing in the United States.

Ask Yourself

Any program of study will require you to commit yourself in many ways, especially in terms of time and energy. As a nurse-midwife-in-training, you will undoubtedly study the human body and fetal development. Additionally, you will learn how to counsel, communicate, and comfort. As you decide if nurse-midwifery is right for you, consider the following questions: Am I excited by the challenge of school? Am I interested in math and science? Do I like working as a part of a team? Do I prefer working for myself? Do I want to work in a hospital?

4

Working as a Nurse-Midwife

Nurse-midwives are not doctors, but they do deliver babies and provide pregnant women with prenatal care. In most states, nurse-midwives can write prescriptions. Additionally, nurse-midwives educate women and their partners about nutrition, exercise, labor, breastfeeding, parent-baby bonding, childcare, and bottle-feeding.

Asking Questions

Nurse-midwives ask a lot of questions. When a pregnant woman comes to see them, they find out about her health. Is she eating properly and getting enough vitamins and minerals? If not, the nurse-midwife prescribes a nutrition plan for the mother-to-be.

They inquire about past illnesses, family health history, previous pregnancies, etc. Developing and maintaining a detailed patient history helps the nurse-midwife make informed and accurate decisions about patient care. The nurse-midwife checks the client's blood pressure and pulse, measures her weight, and performs urine and blood tests, along with any other tests he or she thinks are appropriate. These tests help the nurse-midwife rule out possible infections or illnesses that might affect a pregnant woman and her baby.

Providing Answers

Nurse-midwives also answer a lot of questions. Pregnancy is often a stressful and emotional time for a woman. She will have questions about what is happening to her, both physically and emotionally. She may be nervous about becoming a mother and seek reassurance. A pregnant woman may have questions about whether she should breast-feed or bottle-feed her baby. She will want to know what to expect when she goes into labor. She may have questions about what to do in an emergency.

Nurse-midwives perform prenatal visits in the clinic, hospital, or the family's home. Many women find prenatal visits in their home comforting. During these visits, nurse-midwives find out who will be present at the birth and help the woman develop what is called a birth plan. These visits also allow nurse-midwives time to get to know the patient's family and friends. Some women also prefer to deliver their baby at home. They find the familiar surroundings relaxing.

Well-Woman Care

Nurse-midwives see women who are not pregnant for regular physical examinations or well-woman

Did You Know?

Most nurse-midwives have successful medical practices. On average, nurse-midwives see 140 patients and deliver ten babies each month. In fact, the first study known to examine the risk of infant death during deliveries attended by certified nurse-midwives in the United States shows excellent survival rates for nurse-midwife attended births. The study examined birth records from 1991 and looked at the difference in survival rates between doctor attended and nurse-midwife attended deliveries. Researchers found that the instance of infant death was 19 percent lower in cases when nurse-midwives attended the delivery.

Using a nurse-midwife instead of a doctor has become a more popular and accepted way to have a baby. In a recent study, one woman summed up the type of support she and her family received from her midwife. "A large part of her providing the kind of care we wanted is what she didn't do . . . she didn't rush anything . . . she said to me, 'Your body knows what to do, so just let it do it.'" Overall, women commonly described their midwives as: calm, patient, confident, decisive, intelligent, mature, honest, generous, gentle, and nurturing.

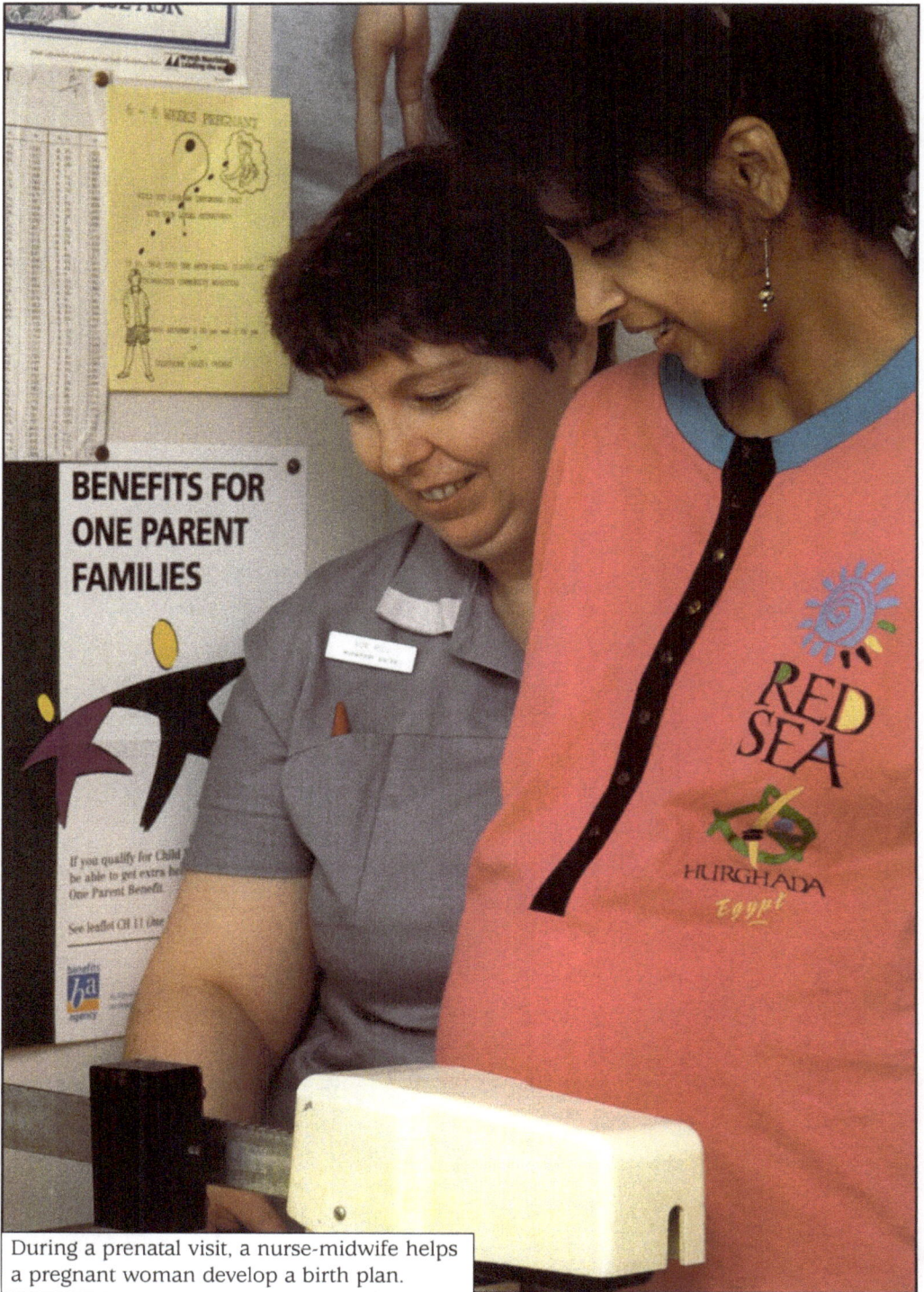

During a prenatal visit, a nurse-midwife helps a pregnant woman develop a birth plan.

care. They help women who are having difficulty getting pregnant by administering tests to determine the nature of the problem. Then, they either treat it themselves or refer their patient to a specialist. They also counsel. They assist their patients who may be in need of treatment for drug or alcohol abuse, financial assistance, or help leaving an abusive relationship.

Teaching

Nurse-midwives teach nurse-midwifery classes. Nurse-midwives also sometimes teach childbirth classes. Many women go to childbirth classes to learn what to expect during labor and delivery. This helps calm their fears. These classes teach breathing techniques to help women relax. Pregnant women also learn different positions that they may find more comfortable when they are in labor. These classes often include films of actual births, so pregnant women can see what happens during delivery.

A Day in the Life of a Nurse-Midwife

Brenda Humber used to be a nurse. She worked with pregnant women in a hospital, but did not enjoy it. "I spent ten hours with a patient in labor and then the doctor would come in at the end and deliver the baby. I felt like I missed all the glory and I wanted more." Brenda went back to school to become a nurse-midwife.

Now, Brenda is a nurse-midwife who shares a private practice with another woman in Illinois. In addition to delivering babies at a nearby hospital, she and her partner see about thirty patients daily. First thing each morning, before setting foot in her office, Brenda goes to the hospital where she makes the rounds, visiting the women whose babies she has delivered. She examines them, answers their questions, and decides when it is time for a mother to return home with her newborn.

Once she finishes rounds at the hospital, she travels to her office. The majority of the patients she sees each day are pregnant. Brenda notes their weight, takes urine and blood samples, discusses nutrition, and monitors the growth and development of the fetus.

Some of Brenda's patients are not pregnant, but they receive regular checkups. During these exams, Brenda may diagnose and treat infections and sexually transmitted diseases, prescribe birth control, and provide overall gynecological care.

Brenda also has an arrangement with an obstetrician, a doctor who deals specifically with childbirth. She refers those patients with potentially complicated pregnancies to this obstetrician. In some cases, these women have illnesses that threaten their pregnancy or perhaps they are having a multiple birth. After a woman sees the obstetrician, the doctor consults Brenda. She and the obstetrician then decide who should continue as the patient's primary care provider. Nursing assistants are also a very important part of Brenda's busy practice. They help administer lab tests and respond to patient questions.

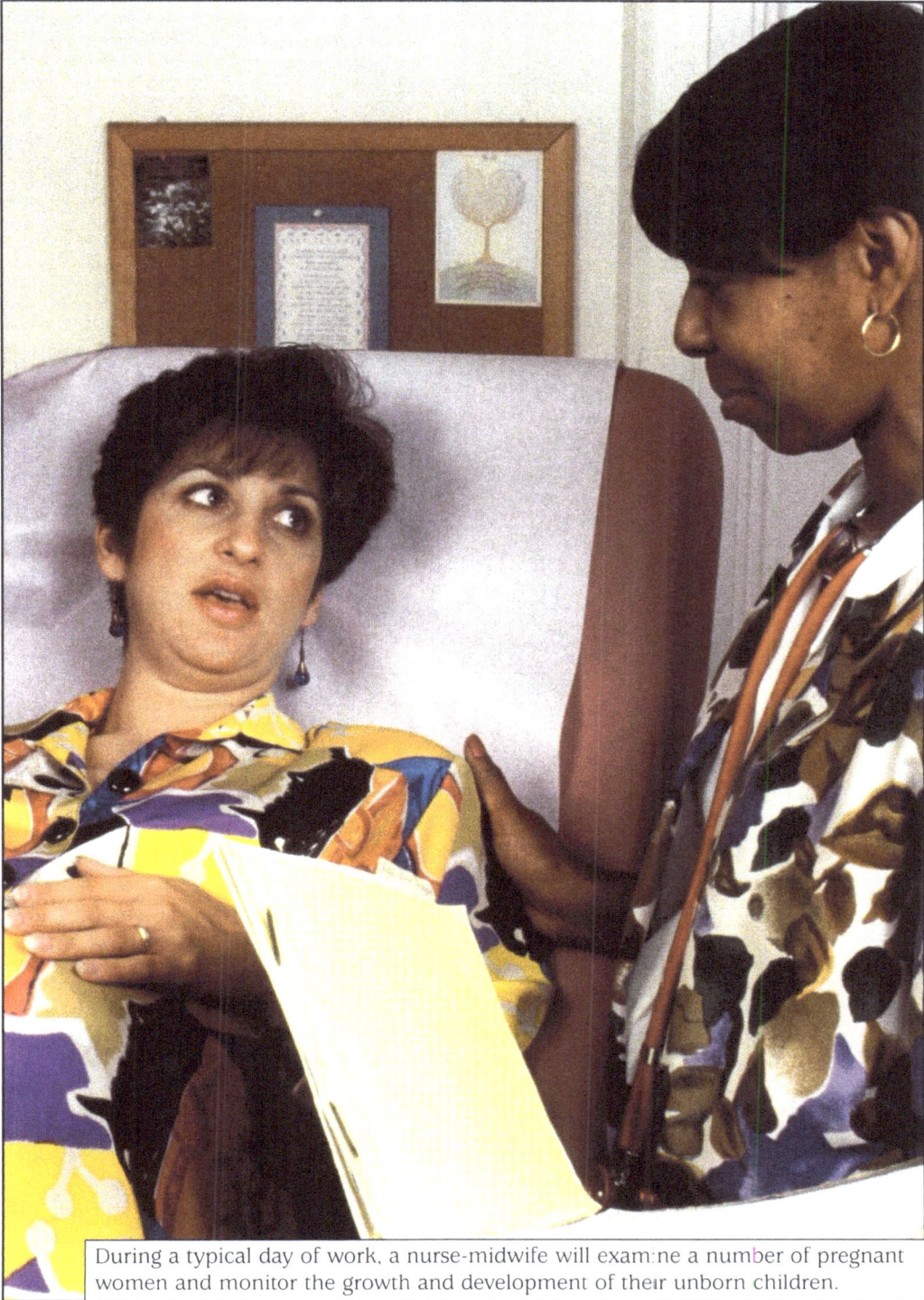

During a typical day of work, a nurse-midwife will examine a number of pregnant women and monitor the growth and development of their unborn children.

Some nights, after Brenda has had a busy day in her office, a mom-to-be in labor awakens her. Brenda then determines if it is time for her patient to go to the hospital, and if so, they meet there. Brenda says, "The downside to midwifery is that you work holidays and miss family functions, but bringing another person into the world, even at 3 AM, outweighs all the bad stuff."

The long hours can also be hard on a nurse-midwife's children and partner. "When my children were young, it was difficult for them to understand that I had to leave to be with someone else's family. But it taught them a maturity and independence they wouldn't have gotten otherwise. Now, they brag to their friends that I'm a midwife."

For Brenda, one of the best aspects of being a nurse-midwife is that she meets people from many different cultures. Also, patients sometimes become a part of her life forever. She often becomes a friend of the women she helps through pregnancy and childbirth. "I become friends with a lot of my patients. For nine months you share some of the most intimate moments of a woman's life," she says. "You see a side of women no one else sees." Brenda believes that being a midwife enables her to have a special relationship with people; one that you cannot find in any other profession. "It's a highly respectful way to treat women," she says. "It is so wonderful that I can't put it into words."

5

A Career with Many Options

One of the advantages of being a nurse-midwife is flexibility. You can decide if you prefer a set work schedule or one that changes day to day. You can also decide where you would prefer to work and in what type of environment you want to care for your clients.

Homes

After having her baby at home in 1974, sociologist Barbara Katz Rothman decided to do a study on nurse-midwives. "I tracked down and interviewed all the people I could find who were attending home-births. All were nurse-midwives." Some had gone through regular nurse training and then moved on to hospital-based midwifery before doing home-births. Some had been trained and worked as midwives before becoming nurse-midwives.

Home-birth can be very different than hospital birth, not only for the birthing woman but also for the person attending. A nurse-midwife can

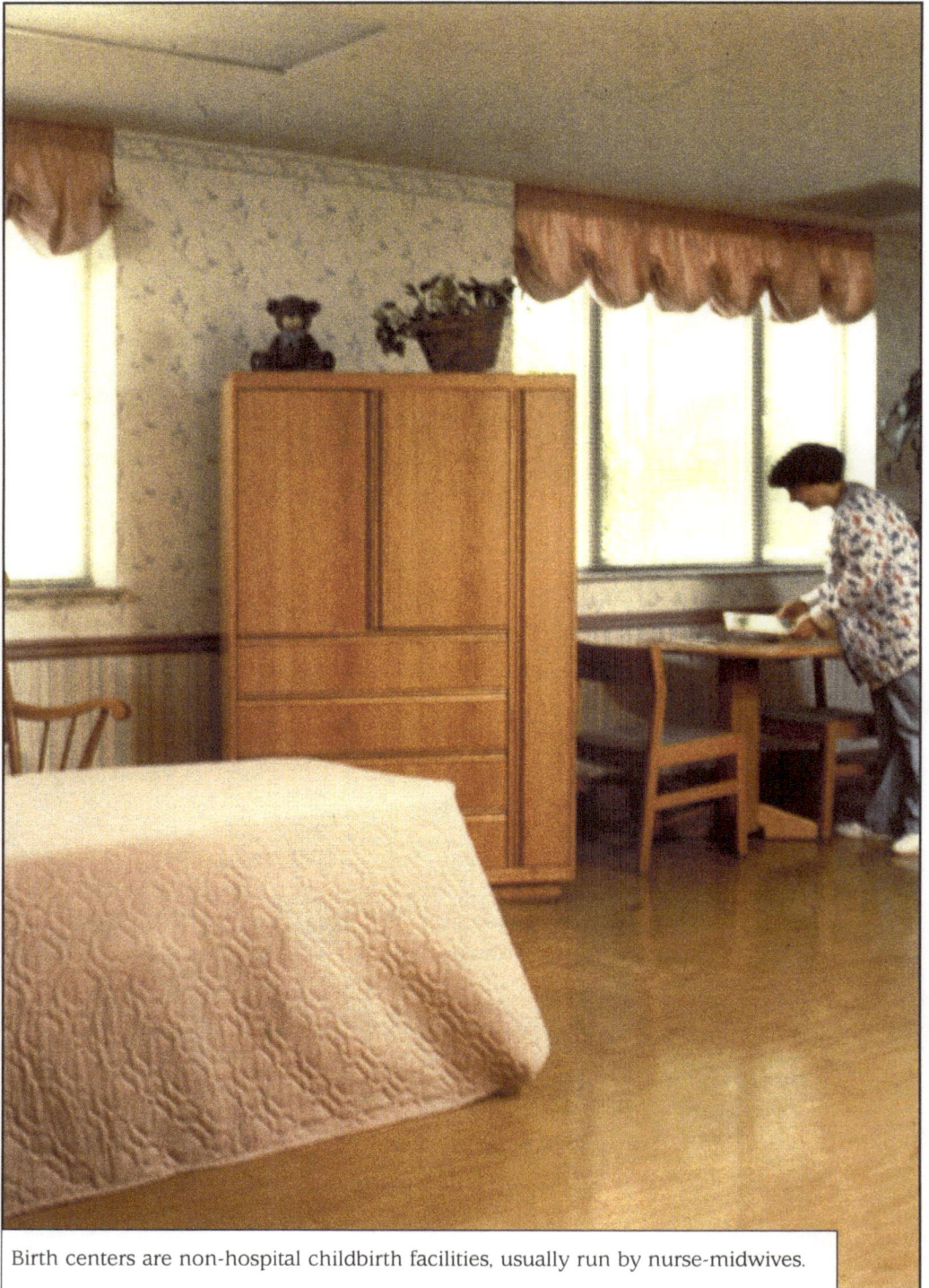

Birth centers are non-hospital childbirth facilities, usually run by nurse-midwives.

bring the hospital way of thinking into the home. A nurse-midwife can also bring the home way of thinking into the hospital. Many nurse-midwives tell stories of doing home-births one day and then doing hospital births the next, trying to take what they had learned at home and applying it in the hospital.

Birth Centers

Birth centers are non-hospital facilities usually run by nurse-midwives, but sometimes by doctors. Here, nurse-midwives see women throughout their pregnancy until they give birth. The same nurse-midwife delivers the baby. Many mothers-to-be prefer this because they are allowed to have anyone they want present for the birth.

Hospitals

Some nurse-midwives work for hospitals. Hospitals are the most popular choice for women when it comes to deciding where to deliver their baby. For many women, a hospital delivery means a safer birth, with access to doctors and medical equipment in case of an emergency.

Some women also choose a hospital because only doctors can administer some medicines for pain. Some nurse-midwives also prefer to work in hospitals, with a routine schedule. Other nurse-midwives dislike the hospital setting because they find themselves delivering the babies of women they did not care for throughout their pregnancy.

Related Professions

Physician

Physicians examine patients, diagnose and treat illnesses, prescribe medicine, and develop a course of treatment. Physicians also perform preventative care like administering immunizations and advising patients about exercise and diet. Many doctors, like nurses, specialize in areas such as obstetrics and pediatrics (caring for children).

After finishing four years of college, physicians must attend medical school for an additional four years. Following medical school, doctors must complete a three-year training program or residency. Sometimes doctors must go to school for a few more years to earn a certificate in their area of specialization. Physicians can earn anywhere from $75,000 to $250,000 per year.

One thing to keep in mind is that the time commitment involved in becoming a physician is tremendous. For instance, an undergraduate who graduates college at the age of twenty-two will most likely finish medical school at twenty-six. Then he or she will perform three years of interning and complete a residency, or training period, at a hospital. At that point, around the age of twenty-nine, the new doctor begins his or her career. Training for some specialties can last until the physician's early to middle thirties. Some people begin their medical education after pursuing other careers, which can further delay the completion of their medical training.

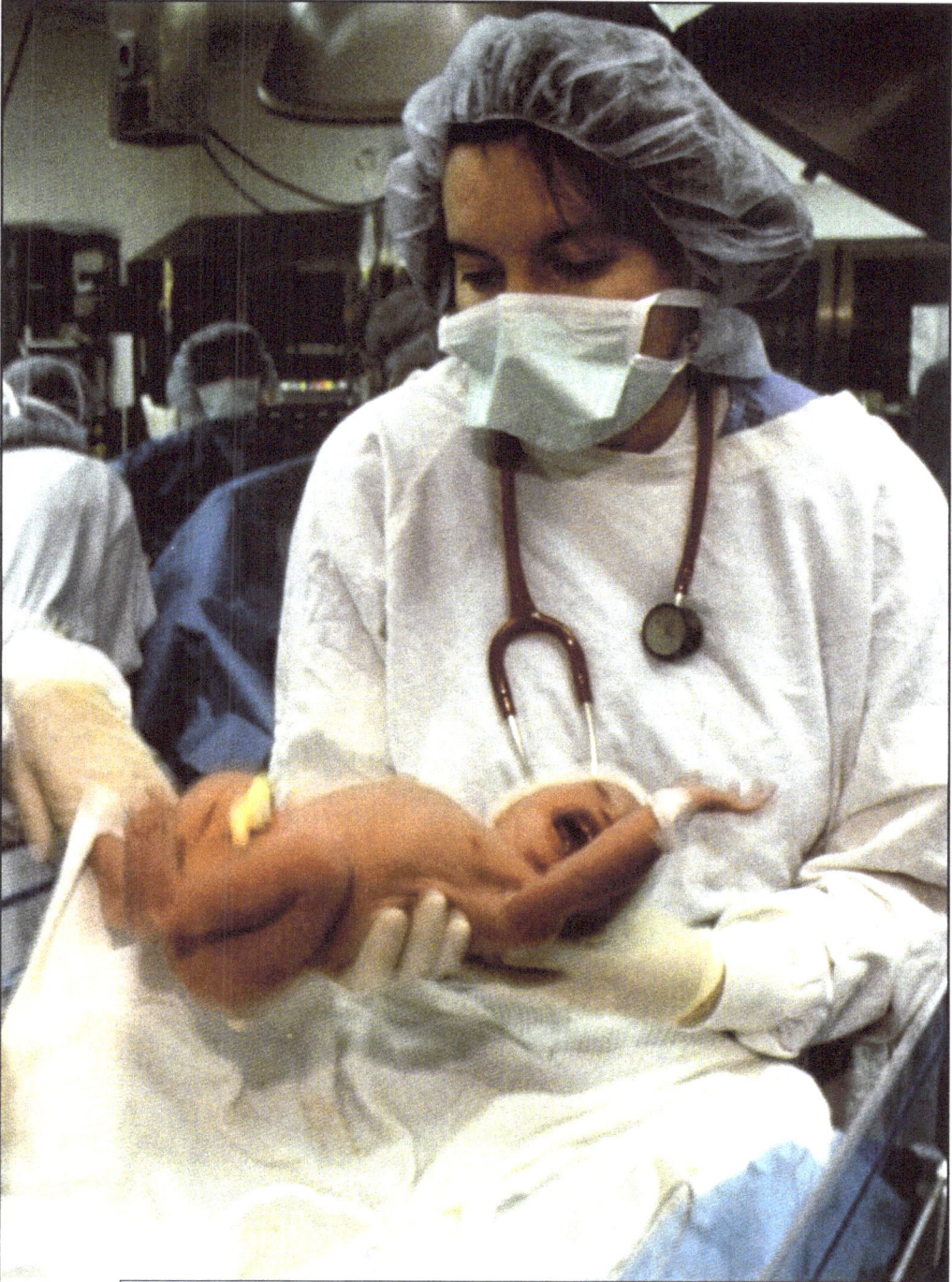

A tremendous time commitment is involved in training to become a physician.

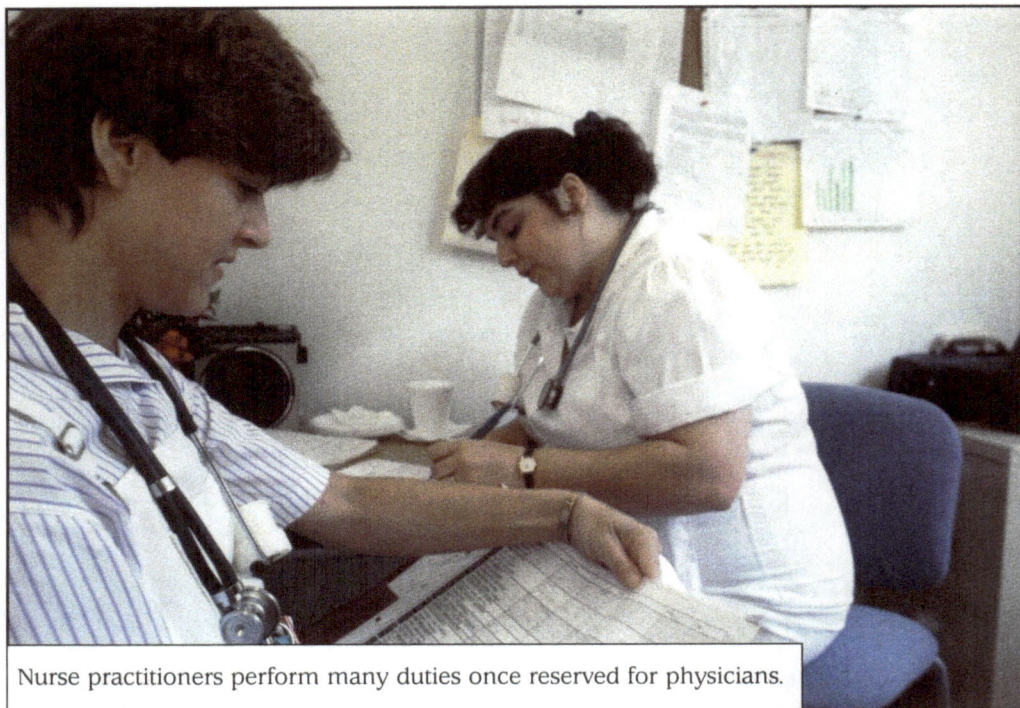

Nurse practitioners perform many duties once reserved for physicians.

Registered Nurse

These nurses provide direct care for sick and injured people. They dress wounds, assist in emergency care, and carry out medical plans prescribed by doctors. They record patient complaints and symptoms. They chart patient reactions to treatment, monitor patient progress, and assist in rehabilitation and recovery.

Nurses may also work as administrators supervising other nurses, or as teachers in a college nursing program. They might also specialize in areas like obstetrics or pediatrics. They work in hospitals, nursing homes, doctor's offices, clinics, and medical centers.

Registered nurses can attend nursing school at a four-year college to earn a bachelor's degree or a two-year college to earn an associate's degree.

Starting annual salary is usually about $30,000. Depending on the level of their education, nurses can eventually earn up to $75,000, especially working as teachers and supervisors.

A registered nurse (RN) must be licensed in order to practice nursing. The National Council of State Boards of Nursing Licensing Exam (NCLEX) is the exam that a graduate nurse must pass in order to become a registered nurse. The new graduate, who is awaiting his or her exam results may work as a graduate nurse (GN) under the direct supervision of a registered nurse.

Nurse Practitioner

These nurses complete not only a nursing program but also an additional nurse practitioner program. They perform nursing duties as well as many tasks once reserved for physicians. They conduct physical examinations, record patient histories, order lab tests, and interpret test results and X rays.

They keep detailed records of their findings, prescribe treatments and therapies, make referrals to doctors, and can even treat many serious illnesses under doctor supervision. They earn anywhere from $48,000 to $80,000 per year. Nurse practitioners can also become teachers and supervisors.

A nurse practitioner is a registered nurse (RN) who has advanced education and clinical training in a health care specialty area. Nurse practitioners work with people of all ages and their families, providing information people need to make informed decisions about their health care. Nurse practitioners practice under the rules and regulations of the Nurse Practice Act of the state in which they work. Most nurse practitioners are also nationally certified in their specialty area. These areas range from emergency care to gynecological care to family practice.

Childbirth Assistant or Doula

Birth assistants, also known as doulas, assist nurse-midwives. The word "doula" comes from the ancient Greek and refers to a trained and experienced woman who provides continuous emotional, physical, and informational support to a woman before, during, and immediately following childbirth. They are often, but not always, nurse-midwives-in-training. Childbirth assistants help the nurse-midwife during both the labor and delivery of the baby. Labor is a very long process and very physically demanding. It is helpful for a nurse-midwife to have an assistant to allow for a break.

The assistant meets the patient toward the end of her pregnancy so that they can become familiar with one another. The assistant gives the patient a list of things she will need to have when it is time to deliver, and may even help the patient learn relaxation techniques for labor.

When a woman goes into labor, the birth assistant may go to the patient's home to encourage the woman to eat, rest, or drink plenty of fluids. The assistant might suggest sitting or standing positions for the woman to relax into that will hopefully make her more comfortable. The assistant also notes the amount of time between contractions and determines when it is time to leave for the hospital or birth center.

The birth assistant remains with a woman throughout labor and delivery. Birth assistants help with the first feedings. Some birth assistants also provide follow-up support to women during their first few days at home.

The benefit of having a doula's support in labor has been recognized by the World Health Organization, the Society of Obstetricians and Gynecologists of Canada, and the Medical Leadership Council, an organization of 1,200 hospitals.

Ask Yourself

Obviously, there are many career options to choose from if you are interested in women's health care and delivering babies. In order to decide what path might be best for you, ask yourself these questions: Do I want to be a nurse who focuses solely on delivering babies? Do I want to be someone who handles medical complications and can perform surgery? Do I like the idea of providing support during labor, but not being entirely responsible for delivering the baby?

Is It Right For You?

Deanne Williams, the current director of the American College of Nurse-Midwives, believes that nurse-midwifery is amazing and gratifying work.

"Nurse-midwifery is very intellectually and emotionally challenging, and often very physically challenging work with many levels of rewards. You have to be smart. You have to be willing to learn. And you have to be willing to keep up with new developments," she says. "You have the ability to have a tremendous impact on the lives of mothers and families in extremely positive ways. I like making a difference in a lot of women's lives, which sometimes means saving lives."

Deanne also encourages people thinking about becoming nurse-midwives to consider the more difficult parts of the job. It is not a job that you perform for only forty hours a week, in your office. Nurse-midwives should be willing to be flexible; babies are not always born on schedule. You often have to get up in the middle of the night. You may have to leave your family on weekends and holidays, or excuse yourself from movies and parties. You can become emotionally tired, so it is important to maintain your own good health to meet these demands.

You should be sensitive. Many women experience a lot of different emotions during pregnancy and you will have to be able to comfort them and encourage them when they need it. Some women who are considering a career as a nurse-midwife may want to start as a childbirth educator or childbirth assistant. Both positions provide an opportunity to watch the birthing process.

You must be willing to be understanding and respectful of your individual patients and their wishes and circumstances. You must be assertive and decisive. You will have the health of others in your hands.

There are many professions to choose from in health care and many things to consider even within nurse-midwifery. Nurse-midwifery provides the opportunity to work closely with women and their families, to bring children into the world, and to teach and train other aspiring nurse midwives. Nurse-midwives are friends and helpers. They are compassionate, intelligent, and caring, and provide help and hope to women everywhere.

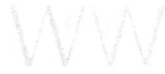

Glossary

birth center   A non-hospital facility where midwives see women throughout their pregnancy right up until they are ready to have the baby. The same midwife will also deliver the baby.

birth plan   A midwife will help a pregnant woman develop a birth plan, which includes where she wants to have the baby and who will be there with her.

breastfeeding   When a woman feeds her baby with the milk she produces from her breasts rather than from a bottle. Some women have difficulty with this and midwives often teach them how to do it.

cesarean   Surgical birth of a baby through the abdomen.

complications   Anything that may happen during labor that is not part of a normal birth. This may include problems with the baby or the mother that require a doctor's intervention or the delivery of the baby through cesarean.

contraction   Labor pain. These can be very painful and can last up to thirty hours. It is necessary for the mother to have these pains to push the baby down and out of her body.

doula   A labor coach and supporter who assists the nurse-midwife with the labor and delivery.

family-centered birth   Most midwives support this type of childbirth, where pregnant women and their families are the focus. The mother-to-be decides how and where her baby will be born and who will be with her.

gynecology   The type of health care that focuses on women's reproductive organs.

high-risk pregnancy   Having a medical condition such as diabetes or high blood pressure or another illness or disease that requires special care during pregnancy and birth. A woman with a high-risk pregnancy may not be able to deliver her baby with a midwife because it may be too dangerous and may require the help of a doctor.

labor   The bodily process that brings the birth of a baby and includes contractions.

nursing assistant   A helper for a nurse or midwife who may work in a private practice or in a hospital. He or she performs some duties for the nurse or midwife, such as taking a patient's temperature, pulse, and blood pressure.

obstetrician   A doctor who treats pregnant women and delivers babies.

prenatal care   The health care a woman receives from a doctor or a midwife while she is pregnant.

For More Information

In the United States

American College of Nurse Midwives (ACNM)
818 Connecticut Avenue NW, Suite 900
Washington, DC 20006
(888) MIDWIFE (643-9433)
(202) 728-9860
Web site: http://www.midwife.org

Association of Labor Assistants and Childbirth
Educators (ALACE)
P.O. Box 382724
Cambridge, MA 02238
(888) 222-5223
(617) 441-2500
Web site: http://server4.hypermart.net/alacehq

California Association of Midwives
Central Office
P.O. Box 460606
San Francisco, CA 94146

(800) 829-5791
Web site: http://www.gst.net/ ~ midwives

Doulas of North America (DONA)
Central Office
13513 North Grove Drive
Alpine, UT 84004
(801) 756-7331
Web site: http://www.dona.com

Midwives Alliance of North America (MANA)
600 Fifth Street
Monett, MO 65708
(888) 923-MANA (6262)
Web site: http://www.mana.org

International Association of Parents and
    Professionals for Safe Alternatives
    in Childbirth (NAPSAC)
Rte. 4, Box 646
Marble Hill, MO 63764-9418
(573) 238-2010
e-mail: napsac@olas.net

In Canada

The Alberta Association of Midwives
Main Post Office
Box 11957
Edmonton, Alberta T5J 3L1
Web site: http://www.agt.net/public/robin1/
    aam_homepage.htm

College of Midwives of British Columbia
Room F503
4500 Oak Street
Vancouver, BC V6H 3N1
Web site: http://www.cmbc.bc.ca/cmbcfram.htm

Midwives Alliance of North America
MANA-CANADA
Box 26141 RPO Sherbrook
Winnipeg, MB R3C 4K9
(888) 923-MANA (6262)
Web site: http://www.mana.org

Ontario Midwifery Consumer Network
P.O. Box 68517
360-A Bloor Street West
Toronto, Ontario M5S 1X1
(416) 410-7075
Web site: http://www.interlog.com/ ~ omcn

For Further Reading

Armstrong, Penny and Sheryl Feldman. *A Midwife's Story*. New York: Arbor House, 1988.

Breckinridge, Mary. *Wide Neighborhoods: A Story of the Frontier Nursing Service*. Lexington, KY: University Press of Kentucky, 1981.

Chester, Penfield, and Sarah Chester McKusik. *Sisters on a Journey: Portraits of American Midwives*. New Brunswick, NJ: Rutgers University Press, 1997.

Cushman, Karen. *The Midwife's Apprentice*. New York: Clarion Books, 1995.

Field, Shelly. *Career Opportunities in Health Care*. New York: Facts on File, 1997.

Gaskin, Ina May. *Spiritual Midwifery*. Summertown, TN: Book Publishing Company, 1990.

Goer, Henci. *The Thinking Woman's Guide to a Better Birth*. New York: Berkeley Publishing Group, 1999.

Hancock, Cheryl. *Health Care Career Starter*. New York: Learning Express, LLC, 1998

Swanson, Barbara. *Careers in Health Care*. Lincoln-wood, IL: VGM Career Horizons, 2000.

Thatcher Ulrich, Laurel. *A Midwife's Tale: The Life of Martha Ballard, Based on Her Diary, 1785–1812.* New York: Vintage Books, 1991.

Van Olphen-Fehr, Juliana. *Diary of a Midwife: The Power of Positive Childbearing.* Westport, CT: Bergin & Garvey, 1998.

Wells, Rosemary. *Mary on Horseback: Three Mountain Stories.* New York: Dial Books for Young Readers, 1998.

Wilson, Robert F. *Careers in Healthcare.* Hauppage, New York: Barron's Education Series, 1999

Index

Acknowledgments

I would like to thank Deanne Williams, Brenda Humber, Michaele Wylde, and Laura Gilbert for their help with this project.

About the Author

Jennifer Fields currently works at *O, The Oprah Magazine* and is a freelance writer living in New York.

Photo Credits

Cover photo © Don Ryan/AP Photo; pp. 2, 38 © Jennie Woodstock; Reflections Photolibrary/Corbis; p. 7 © James Marshall/Corbis; pp. 9, 47 © Annie Griffiths Belt/Corbis; pp. 11, 13 © SuperStock; pp. 17, 23 © Archive Photos; pp. 18, 21 © Corbis/Bettmann-UPI; p. 24 © AP Photo/*The Chronicle*, Toni L. Baily; p. 28 © Associated Press/AP; p. 32 © Pictor; p. 44 © Mike Moreland/Custom Medical Stock Photo; p. 48 © Robert Maass/Corbis.

Design

Geri Giordano

Layout

Les Kanturek

www.ingramcontent.com/pod-product-compliance
Lightning Source LLC
Chambersburg PA
CBHW061152030426
42336CB00002B/23